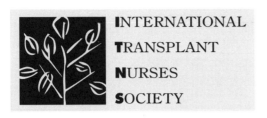

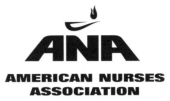

TRANSPLANT NURSING:
SCOPE AND STANDARDS
OF PRACTICE

D1568474

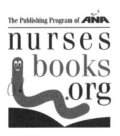

The Publishing Program of ANA
nurses
books
.org

INTERNATIONAL TRANSPLANT NURSES SOCIETY

AMERICAN NURSES ASSOCIATION
SILVER SPRING, MARYLAND
2009

Library of Congress Cataloging-in-Publication data

Transplant nursing : scope and standards of practice / International Transplant Nurses Society.
   p. ; cm.
   Includes bibliographical references and index.
   ISBN-13: 978-1-55810-266-8 (softcover : alk. paper)
   ISBN-10: 1-55810-266-3 (softcover : alk. paper)
   1. Transplantation of organs, tissues, etc—Nursing. I. American Nurses Association. II. Title.
   [DNLM: 1. Nursing—standards. 2. Organ Transplantation—nursing. 3. Clinical Competence—standards. 4. Nursing Care—standards. WY 161 I61 2009]
   RD129.8.I68 2009
   617.9′5—dc22   2009015754

The American Nurses Association (ANA) is a national professional association. This ANA publication—*Transplant Nursing: Scope and Standards of Practice*—reflects the thinking of the nursing profession on various issues and should be reviewed in conjunction with state board of nursing policies and practices. State law, rules, and regulations govern the practice of nursing, while *Transplant Nursing: Scope and Standards of Practice* guides nurses in the application of their professional skills and responsibilities.

The International Transplant Nurses Society (ITNS) is a non-profit organization committed to promoting the education and clinical practice excellence of nurses who are interested and participate in the care of solid organ transplant patients. Founded in 1992, ITNS offers nurses a forum for sharing and learning about the latest advances in transplantation and transplant patient care with national and international peers. It provides, promotes, and supports educational and professional growth opportunities, interprofessional networking and collaborative activities, and research in transplant clinical nursing. ITNS website: http://itns.org

Published by Nursesbooks.org
The Publishing Program of ANA

American Nurses Association
8515 Georgia Avenue, Suite 400
Silver Spring, MD 20910-3492
1-800-274-4ANA
http://www.Nursesbooks.org/

The ANA is the only full-service professional organization representing the interests of the nation's 2.9 million registered nurses through its 53 constituent member nurses associations and its 24 specialty nursing and workforce advocacy affiliate organizations that currently connect to ANA as affiliates. The ANA advances the nursing profession by fostering high standards of nursing practice, promoting the rights of nurses in the workplace, projecting a positive and realistic view of nursing, and by lobbying the Congress and regulatory agencies on health care issues affecting nurses and the public.

Design: Scott Bell, Arlington, VA ~ Freedom by Design, Alexandria, VA ~ Stacy Maguire, Sterling, VA ~ *Editorial Management*: Eric Wurzbacher, ANA ~ *Copyediting*: Steven Jent, Denton, TX ~ *Proofreading*: Ashley Mason, Atlanta GA ~ *Indexing*: Estalita Slivoskey, Havre de Grace, MD ~ *Composition*: House of Equations, Inc., Arden, NC ~ *Printing*: Linemark Printing, Inc., Upper Marlboro, MD

First printing May 2009.

ISBN-13: 978-1-55810-266-8   SAN: 851-3481   2.5M   05/09

ACKNOWLEDGMENTS

This scope and standards of transplant nursing practice document was created by a task force from the International Transplant Nurses Society (ITNS). This diverse group of transplant nurses was instrumental in developing this document. Many thanks to Carol J. Bickford, PhD, RN-BC, Senior Policy Fellow, American Nurses Association Department of Nursing Practice and Policy, for her support and expertise in guiding the development of this specialty nursing scope and standards of practice.

Scope and Standards Task Force Members

Patricia G. Folk, RN, BSN, CCTC

Cindy Hoekstra, RN, BScN, CCTN

Evelyn Jirasakhiran, RN, MS

Beth Kallenborn, RN, BSN, CCTC

Beverly Kosmach-Park, MSN, CRNP

Darlene Long, MS, APRN, BC, ANP, CCTC

Sandra Martin, RN, MSN

Moira Perrin, RGN, BSc(Honors)

Bonnie Potter, RN, CCTC

Wanda Ryan, RN, C, CCTC

Barb Schroeder, MS, RN, CNS

Kathy Schwab, RN, BSN, CCTC

Tammy Sebers, RN, BSN, CNN

Frank VanGelder, RN, BSN, ECTC

Anneloes Wilschut, RN, CCRN

Cynthia L. Russell, PhD, RN, APRN, BC *(Chair)*

Scope and Standards Reviewers

Sandra Cupples, PhD, RN

Sabina De Geest, PhD, RN, FAAN, FRCN

Donna Hathaway, PhD, RN, FAAN

Linda Ohler, RN, MSN, CCTC, FAAN

Melissa Inglese, PhD, MSN, RN

Scope and Standards Participating Organization

International Transplant Nurses Society

American Nurses Association (ANA) Staff

Carol J. Bickford, PhD, RN-BC

Yvonne Humes, MSA – Project coordinator

Maureen E. Cones, Esq. – Legal counsel

CONTENTS

Scope and Standards of Transplant Nursing Practice

Function of the Scope of Practice Statement

The scope of practice statement (pages 1–22) describes the "who", "what", "where", "when", "why" and "how" of nursing practice. Each of these questions must be sufficiently answered to provide a complete picture of the practice and its boundaries and membership. The depth and breadth in which individual registered nurses engage in the total scope of nursing practice is dependent upon education, experience, role, and the population served.

Function of Standards

The Standards, which are comprised of the standards of practice (pages 23–36) and the standards of professional performance (pages 37–47), are authoritative statements by which nurses practicing within the role, population, and specialty governed by this document (*Transplant Nursing: Scope and Standards of Practice*) and that describe the duties that they are expected to competently perform. The Standards published herein may be utilized as evidence of the legal standard of care governing nurses practicing within the role, population, and specialty governed by this document. The Standards are subject to change with the dynamics of the nursing profession and as new patterns of professional practice are developed and accepted by the nursing profession and the public. In addition, specific conditions and clinical circumstances may also affect the application of the Standards at a given time; e.g., during a natural disaster. The Standards are subject to formal, periodic review and revision.

The measurement criteria that appear below each standard are not all-inclusive and do not establish the legal standard of care. Rather, the measurement criteria are specific, measurable elements that can be used by nursing professionals to measure professional performance. Nurses practicing within this particular role, population, and specialty can identify opportunities for development and improvement by evaluating performance on these elements.

Scope of Transplant Nursing Practice

Function of the Scope of Practice Statement

The scope of practice statement (pages 1–22) describes the "who", "what", "where", "when", "why" and "how" of nursing practice. Each of these questions must be sufficiently answered to provide a complete picture of the practice and its boundaries and membership. The depth and breadth in which individual registered nurses engage in the total scope of nursing practice is dependent upon education, experience, role, and the population served.

Introduction to Transplant Nursing

Solid organ transplantation offers the best treatment option for improved quality of life for people of all ages with end-stage solid organ disease (Galbraith & Hathaway, 2004). Since the first successful kidney transplant was performed in 1954, solid organ transplantation has continued to advance as a treatment for end-stage organ diseases of the kidney, pancreas, liver, heart, lung, and small bowel.

The number of transplants worldwide continues to grow. The number of transplants completed in the United States in 1988 was 12,623. By 2007, the number had risen to 28,357. The number of individuals needing an organ continues to increase dramatically with the growing number of individuals with diseases such as diabetes and cardiovascular disease resulting in organ failure. The demand for solid organs for transplantation is greater than the number of donor organs available (UNOS, 2008). Though living donation has expanded over the last 50 years to include other organs (e.g., liver and lung), the need for solid organs from both living and deceased donors continues to escalate.

The recent 50-year anniversary of the first successful transplant has drawn attention to the contribution of nursing to the success of transplantation. Multiple factors influence the provision of transplant nursing care. Transplant patients require specialized care based upon expert knowledge and skills from experienced transplant nurses. As the acuity of transplant patients increases and the length of hospitalization after transplantation decreases, transplant nurses are required to provide high-level, expanded care to patients and their families outside the traditional hospital setting.

Advancing technology and treatments require transplant nurses to make a lifelong commitment to learning. Organ shortages require that transplant nurses help educate the community about the need to donate. Providing collaborative care as members of interprofessional teams of specialists is just one of the roles of transplant nurses. The global shortage of nurses in general, and transplant nurses in particular, continues to grow, and the transplant nurse will be challenged to provide the best care to transplant patients with limited resources. The population continues to live longer both with and without a transplant. Consequently, individuals must live many years with multiple chronic illnesses.

In the midst of these circumstances and changes, the transplant nurse continues to provide specialized care to patients, their families, and communities, blending the science and art of nursing. The nurse's role and function is differentiated according to education, position description, and practice setting, with these factors further defining practice. Nursing education varies widely throughout the world; nursing practice varies dramatically as well. Because each country, state, and province has its own laws regulating nursing, the limits, functions, and titles for nurses may differ from state to state and country to country, particularly at the advanced practice level. Nurses must ensure that their practice remains within the boundaries defined by their governmental agencies. However, transplant nurses must continually examine their practice, looking for ways to improve the practice of nursing throughout the world.

This document addresses the role, scope, and standards of nursing practice for the specialty of transplant nursing. The scope of practice addresses the definition of transplant nursing, its various levels of practice based on educational preparation recognizing its worldwide variations, current clinical practice activities and sites, and current evidence-based practice relevant to transplant nursing. The standards of transplant nursing practice are objective, measurable statements of the responsibilities for which transplant nurses are accountable.

Solid organ transplantation is distinct from bone marrow transplantation, which treats diseases of the blood. Nursing care provided to bone marrow transplant recipients is covered in such publications as *Statement on the Scope and Standards of Advanced Practice Nursing in Oncology* (3rd Edition) from the Oncology Nursing Society (ONS) and *Pediatric Oncology Nursing: Scope and Standards of Practice* from the Association of Pediatric Hematology/Oncology Nurses (APHON).

Description of Transplant Nursing

Transplant nursing is specialized nursing care focused on protection, promotion, and optimization of the health and abilities of both the transplant recipient and the living donor across the life span. This care includes prevention, detection, and treatment of illness and injury related to diseases treated by solid organ transplantation, and diseases that may result from living donor donation in individuals, families, communities, and populations of all ages.

Transplant nursing is also specialized nursing care focused on protection, promotion, and optimization of the deceased organ donor and the living organ donor during the process of organ donation. This care includes prevention, detection, and treatment of illness and injury that may occur during the process of organ donation and recovery in individuals and families of all ages.

Transplant nursing encompasses care and support of the ill organ recipient or potential recipient who may have multi-organ and multi-system disease processes, the deceased donor, and the healthy person who desires to donate or has donated an organ. Transplant nursing requires knowledge of immunology, transplant pharmacology, infectious diseases, and psychological implications of caring for the morbidity and mortality faced by the potential transplant recipient, the organ donor, and their families and communities. In communities, transplant nurses provide organ donation support and education. Transplant nursing is the application of evidence-based care to individuals, families, and communities through all phases of the transplant process to optimize health, functional ability, and quality of life. This care includes assisting individuals of all ages, and their families and communities, with the transplant processes that may affect their lives.

Key Elements

Key elements of transplant nursing include:

- Patient education;
- Interventions that maintain or improve physiologic, psychological, and social health;
- Interventions that facilitate and optimize behavioral change and treatment adherence with complex, lifelong therapies;
- Advocacy to support patients and families in the planning, implementation, and evaluation of their care; and
- System improvements to support optimal transplant outcomes.

Once a transplant or living donation occurs, transplant nurses continue to promote optimal health, disease and injury prevention, symptom recognition, disease management, and alleviation of suffering in individuals, families, and communities.

Transplant nursing also encompasses the optimization of the system in which transplant care is delivered. These aspects of care center on quality monitoring, collaboration, education, research, and administration. Other key elements of nursing care provided by transplant nurses include development, initiation, and maintenance of systems and processes that promote teamwork, collaboration, efficiency, and patient satisfaction. Transplant nursing is based on health provider education, patient safety, and care efficacy.

Research

The relatively new area of transplant nursing research broadens the knowledge base of transplant nursing care. The dimensions of practice described above are just now beginning to be systematically tested through transplant nursing research. The International Transplant Nurses Society (ITNS) promotes transplant research and evidence-based practice by providing several research grants each year. The recipients disseminate their findings through the ITNS annual symposium and publications. There are many opportunities for research because transplant care is diverse and often specific to a given institution in which transplant care is provided.

Practice Settings and Roles

The transplant nurse works in a variety of settings, which may include the wards or units, intensive care units, and operating rooms of hospitals, ambulatory care clinics, other clinical facilities, and the community. The transplant nurse may concentrate on:

- Clinical care (as a *clinical nurse*),
- Coordination of care (as a *transplant nurses coordinator*):
  - for the transplant recipient (as a *recipient nurse coordinator*),
  - for the deceased donor (as a *procurement nurse coordinator*),
  - for the living donor (as a *living donor nurse coordinator*), or
- Advanced clinical care (as an *advanced practice transplant nurse*).

The clinical nurse works in patient care wards or units, operating rooms, and clinics. The transplant nurse coordinator and advanced practice transplant nurse also work in a multitude of settings such as inpatient units, and outpatient clinics, providing direct patient care, coordinating all aspects of care, and providing support through education and research.

The procurement nurse coordinator often works in the intensive care environment and operating rooms, but may also travel to distant centers to provide patient and staff education and to assist with procurement of organs. Following donation efforts, the procurement nurse coordinator has a significant role in providing follow-up support and advocacy for donor families, often by phone or other electronic communications.

The living donor nurse coordinator works predominantly in clinics to prepare and educate donors about donating their organs. Following donation, the living donor nurse coordinator will follow patients for varying lengths of time to enhance recovery and continued health.

The transplant nurse coordinator, regardless of practice setting or concentration, is an ambassador for organ donation and transplantation and as such also has a role in education at public events, hospitals, and schools.

The table on the following page summarizes the nursing care focus of each of these roles. A more detailed discussion of the transplant nurse

Transplant Nursing Roles and Foci of Nursing Care

Types of transplant nursing roles	Focus of nursing care
Clinical nurse	Transplant clinical care for the transplant plant patient, organ donor, and/or family
Recipient nurse coordinator	Coordination of care for transplant recipient
Procurement nurse coordinator	Pre-donation care, organ procurement, support for deceased donor family
Living donor nurse coordinator	Pre- and post-donation care of living donor
Advance practice transplant nurse	Leadership and advanced transplant clinical care

coordinator begins on page 10, and of the advanced practice transplant nurse begins on page 13.

Development of Transplant Nursing Practice

Growth of Transplant Care and Transplant Nursing

Since the first kidney transplant over 50 years ago, transplant nursing practice has continued to evolve. Advances in transplantation care include improvements in transplant pharmacology, development of new transplant technology, and new surgical procedures to transplant other solid organs. The scope of nursing practice initially involved providing hospital- and community-based transplant care to individuals and families experiencing acute, chronic, and critical illnesses requiring transplantation, and deceased and living donors. The scope of practice has expanded to include people awaiting transplant in the hospital or community with life-supporting technology bridging them to transplantation, those living with a transplanted organ for many years, patients who are re-transplanted, and living donors after they have donated organs.

The current practice of transplant nursing requires extensive clinical knowledge and expertise to provide highly specialized acute, critical, or end-of-life care to hospitalized patients. The practice has also expanded to include increased emphasis on organ donation through the education of individuals, families, communities, and other healthcare providers. Transplant nurses collaborate with individuals, families, communities, and other healthcare professionals to encourage patient self-care using symptom and disease management in order to improve patient outcomes.

Significant advances in transplant care for people who donate a solid organ or who receive a transplant create a need for many roles, such as caregivers, coordinators, educators, administrators, care managers, and quality specialists who optimize transplant outcomes. Transplant nurses manage and provide unique, complex treatments to donor and transplant patients. For example, the person receiving a heart and kidney transplant because of complications from diabetes mellitus will require patient education related to physiology, pathophysiology, self-monitoring, follow-up appointments, testing and lab results, medications, role changes, and safety. The transplant nurse must be knowledgeable to teach individuals and families about complex topics (physiology, pathophysiology, signs and symptoms to monitor, when to contact the transplant team, diet, exercise, role changes, and medications). The transplant nurse must also educate and support the patient's caregiver. As transplant technology expands, caregivers are frequently required to provide home-based support and advanced care for someone who is awaiting or has received a transplant.

The transplant nurse seeks to go beyond the general nursing role of one who cares for a patient who happens to have a transplant. Instead, the transplant nurse demonstrates a strong interest in caring for individuals who have had a transplant or for those who are donating an organ, a desire to improve care for this unique population, and a love for lifelong learning related to transplant nursing. To be a transplant nurse requires a level of transplant nursing knowledge (basic or advanced) and transplant care nursing skills that are setting-specific and that include assessment, diagnosis, planning, implementation, and evaluation of transplant care that attains, maintains, or restores health or leads to a peaceful death. Transplant nursing roles have expanded to include more autonomous actions, including the development of advanced practice nursing roles such as the clinical nurse specialist and nurse practitioner.

International Transplant Nurses Society (ITNS)

There are many transplant organizations available to assist the transplant nurse with continuing education and professional growth. However, transplant nurses are represented by the International Transplant Nurses Society (ITNS). ITNS serves the educational and professional needs of over 1,700 transplant nurses. ITNS was founded in 1992 as an organization committed to the promotion of excellence in transplant clinical nursing through the provision of educational and professional growth opportunities, interprofessional networking and collaborative activities, and transplant nursing research. Twenty-six national and international local chapters have been chartered; they promote the field of transplant nursing through their geographical region and transplant centers.

The goals of ITNS are to:

- Provide a network for communication among professional transplant nurses.
- Provide a means of continuing education for professional transplant nurses.
- Examine new trends in transplantation affecting patient care and the role of the transplant nurse.
- Promote and support research in transplant nursing.
- Distribute the results of scientific investigations among professionals interested in transplantation.
- Foster an awareness of ongoing ethical considerations in procurement, donation, and recipient care.
- Ensure the accomplishment of the proper and lawful purposes and objectives of the society.

In addition, the ITNS through its board of directors is committed to the field of transplantation and strives to maintain the mission and integrity of the society through its activities and educational collaborations. ITNS promotes transplant research and evidence-based practice by providing several research grants each year. The grant recipients disseminate their findings through the ITNS annual symposium and publications. ITNS promotes adherence and patient self management through the publication of patient education brochures on a variety of post-transplant problems (diabetes, skin cancer, gingival hyperplasia, gastrointestinal complications, etc.) and strategies for maintaining a healthy lifestyle following transplantation.

Consequently, ITNS has developed the first scope and standards of practice for transplant nurses and sought specialty nursing recognition from the American Nurses Association. This document will provide a foundation for transplant nursing that will require ongoing review and revision as the state of the art and science of transplant nursing continues to evolve.

Practice Characteristics: Collaboration and Role Differentiation

Nurses working in the field of transplantation specialize their transplant practice in the realm of either donor or recipient care, but not both. The goal of role differentiation is to enhance donor and recipient advocacy and confidentiality, and to reduce conflict of interest.

The integrative nature of transplantation requires the nurse to collaborate daily with members of the interprofessional team to provide comprehensive, ethical, and evidence-based care. In all realms of transplant nursing, the nurse is an advocate for organ donation and transplantation, working to increase awareness among healthcare professionals and the community. Roles of the transplant nurse may include, but are not limited to: clinical nurse, transplant nurse coordinator, educator, case manager, counselor, patient advocate, consultant, researcher, administrator, and advanced practice registered nurse.

The clinical nurse provides nursing care to the transplant patient, organ donor, or family. The roles of transplant nurse coordinator are similar to case management, but in transplant care has three distinct roles:

- The procurement nurse coordinator and the living donor nurse coordinator manage all aspects of the donation process and long-term follow up.
- The recipient nurse coordinator provides care to the patient who will receive a transplanted organ.

Other characteristics common to and different between the practice of these nurse coordinators are summarized on pages 10–12 and described further on pages 14–15.

Transplant Nurse Coordinator

While the role of *transplant nurse coordinator* is unique to transplantation, it is similar to a case manager in its role diversity. Most transplant coordinators, wherever they practice around the world, are registered nurses, but they may be licensed as other healthcare providers, for instance paramedics. The transplant nurse coordinator:

- Has extensive experience in nursing and transplantation,
- Has a global transplant nursing perspective with a focus on a patient's long-term goals,
- Learns from experience what to expect in a given situation and alters plans accordingly,
- Has an intuitive grasp of situations and operates from a deep understanding of the situation,
- Recognizes when situations are outside the expected and uses analytical skills and abilities to investigate alternative perspectives,
- Conducts comprehensive assessments,
- Promotes health and the prevention of injury and disease,
- Serves as an advocate and educator for patient and family,
- Provides consultation and education to healthcare providers and the community regarding transplant issues, and
- Participates in research to improve transplant nursing practice.

Procurement Nurse Coordinator

The *procurement nurse coordinator* ensures compassionate and confidential care for all deceased donors and their families, allowing them to fulfill their final wish to donate the gift of life. The procurement nurse coordinator's care includes, but is not limited to:

- Assessment and management of physiological processes of the deceased donor.
- Teaching deceased donor families about the donation process.
- Providing emotional support to the deceased donor family during the donation process.
- Coordinating the process of organ removal, and allocation to the recipient.

Living Donor Nurse Coordinator

The *living donor nurse* coordinator works with people who wish to donate an organ to ensure they are fully prepared for their experience, evaluated, and followed closely long-term to optimize outcomes. The living donor nurse coordinator's care includes such responsibilities as:

- Assessment and management of the living donor's emotional response to donation.

- Management of the living donor's goals and outcomes of donation.

- Management of the financial impact on the living donor.

- Follow-up of the long-term health of the donor.

Recipient Nurse Coordinator

The *recipient nurse coordinator* provides care to the patient who will receive a transplanted organ, both before and after transplantation.

Pre-transplant care – The recipient nurse coordinator focuses on managing issues related to organ failure to ensure the patient remains in optimal health, enabling the patient to proceed with transplantation once a suitable organ is available. The recipient nurse coordinator's pre-transplant care includes, but is not limited to:

- Managing the potential recipient's evaluation to determine whether that person is a candidate for transplant.

- Assessing and managing the candidate's health so that when transplantation is imminent, the candidate is in optimal physiological, psychological, and psychosocial health.

- Assisting the candidate to cope with the potentially long wait to receive a transplant.

- Providing anticipatory teaching about such post-transplant issues as self-monitoring and reporting, infections, rejections, cancer, medications (cost, number, side effects), intensity and frequency of contact with transplant team, and return to pre-transplant activities.

Post-transplant care – The recipient transplant nurse coordinator helps the patient to achieve the highest level of wellness possible. The nurse's post-transplant care includes such activities as providing:

- Emotional support (e.g., acceptance of feelings of guilt in receiving an organ from someone has undergone surgery or died).

- Patient education related to such post-transplant issues as self-monitoring and reporting, signs of infection and rejection, increased potential for later cancer diagnosis, complex and long-term medication schedules and treatment adherence, intensity and frequency of contact with transplant team, and return to pre-transplant activities.

Generalist Level Transplant Nursing

The transplant nurse working at the generalist level delivers specific services on a routine basis to patients and their families. A registered nurse license or international equivalent is required. At a minimum, the transplant nurse practicing at the generalist level must obtain education, clinical experience, and ongoing continuing education as recommended for all nurses. Preparatory courses are offered to the nurse who wants to specialize in transplantation, or the nurse may receive formal or informal institution-specific training under the supervision of an experienced transplant nurse. Transplant nursing practice at the generalist level includes, but is not limited to, assessment, diagnosis, outcomes identification, plan of care, interventions, and evaluation of care.

Advanced Practice Transplant Nursing

Advanced Practice Registered Nurse

The *advanced practice registered nurse* (APRN) is "a registered nurse who has acquired the expert knowledge base, complex decision-making skills, and clinical competencies for expanded practice, the characteristics of which are shaped by the context and/or country in which s/he is credentialed to practice. A master's degree is recommended for entry level" (ICN, 2002).

In transplant nursing, the APRN functions in the position of nurse practitioner or clinical nurse specialist. Some countries require graduation from an approved school of nursing for advanced practice but may or may not require a registered nursing license. The advanced practice roles include, but are not limited to:

- Specialized and expanded knowledge and skills,

- Advanced assessment and ability to synthesize data and interventions, and

- Significant role autonomy, with the integration and application of a broad range of theoretical and evidence-based knowledge.

The overall role of the APRN in transplant nursing is to provide leadership and advanced clinical expertise to promote optimal patient outcomes and further the growth of transplant nursing at the institutional, national, and international levels. Although the scopes of practice for nurses and advanced practice registered nurses are distinctly different, they do share some transplant knowledge and skills.

Nurse Practitioner

The *nurse practitioner* (NP) specializing in transplant care is a nurse who has completed advanced nursing preparation at the master's or doctoral level. The role requires expanded knowledge and skills for providing expert care to individuals or populations needing transplantation. The NP is skilled in formulating a differential diagnosis. The NP combines patient assessment findings with scientific and clinical knowledge, considers such factors as the behavioral sciences, health and illness experiences, pathophysiology, psychopathology, epidemiology, infectious diseases, clinical manifestations of acute illness, chronic disease, emergency health needs, and normal health events, and uses these skills to diagnose illness and disease.

Collaboration and consultations with other disciplines help provide targeted health services that meet individual patients' needs according to evidence-based practice, scientific rationale, and evidence-based guidelines. From the differential diagnosis through the physical exam, diagnostic and laboratory investigations, the NP provides pharmacologic and non-pharmacologic treatments for the management and treatment of acute and chronic illness and disease. The NP's practice demonstrates strong health promotion and prevention of illness and complications in the transplant recipient's care. The NP can be found in primary, acute, and long-term settings, and practices both autonomously and in collaboration with other healthcare professionals to treat and manage health problems related to transplantation. The NP serves in a variety of settings as patient advocate for individuals, families, groups, and communities, and as a researcher and a consultant.

Clinical Nurse Specialist

The *clinical nurse specialist* (CNS) in transplant care is a nurse who has completed nursing preparation at the master's or doctoral level as a CNS. The CNS is a clinical expert who works with patients and their families, the healthcare team, and the organization (NACNS, 2004). As an expert in evidence-based transplant nursing practice, the CNS treats and manages the health problems of transplant patients and populations. The CNS practices autonomously, integrating knowledge of disease and medical conditions into the prevention, assessment, diagnosis, and treatment of patients' illnesses. The CNS works collaboratively with other members of the healthcare team. The CNS designs, implements, and evaluates both patient-specific and population-based programs of care. The CNS in transplantation acts a leader by advancing the practice of transplant nursing to achieve quality and cost-effective patient outcomes, and guiding interprofessional groups to design and implement innovative solutions to systems and patient care problems. As a direct care provider, the CNS in transplantation performs comprehensive health assessments, forms differential diagnoses, and in some states and countries may have prescriptive authority to prescribe pharmacologic and non-pharmacologic treatments for the direct management and treatment of acute and chronic illness and disease. The CNS in transplantation serves as the patient advocate and educator, provides expert consultation and education to healthcare providers, and conducts and interprets research to improve practice.

Specialty Certification for Transplant Nurses

The transplant nurse can further demonstrate commitment to improving the quality of nursing care by pursuing certification in the field of transplantation. Currently, there are numerous recognized transplant certification programs around the world. The transplant nurse who has the necessary knowledge and skills to care for transplant donors and recipients may validate this competency by taking the certification examination. The following certifications are available:

- Certified Clinical Transplant Nurse,
- Certified Clinical Transplant Coordinator, and
- Certified Procurement Transplant Coordinator.

The transplant nurse must be active in maintaining knowledge and competence at all levels. The nurse is responsible to reflect on and assess daily practice to identify knowledge deficits or areas for improvement. The nurse must work within the identified scopes of practice. Standards of practice for the profession and the specialty guide daily practice.

Educational Requirements for Transplant Nurses

A state, commonwealth, territory, government, or other regulatory body provides an established mechanism for recognition and authorization of adequately educated and prepared individuals to practice nursing, including the specialty of transplant nursing. The associated registration or licensing processes vary from country to country. A nurse in the United States (U.S.) is licensed by a state and is called a registered nurse. The individual is educationally prepared for competent practice at the beginning level upon graduation from an approved U.S. school of nursing and then becomes qualified by examination for registered nurse licensure. Some countries require graduation from an approved school of nursing but may or may not require a registered nursing license. Other countries, such as Germany, require the nurse take a state examination after three years of education.

New nurses may enter the profession with a variety of educational degrees. Experienced nurses become proficient in one or more practice areas or roles, and may focus on patient care in clinical nursing practice specialties, including transplant nursing. Specialized transplant nursing knowledge and experiences may be acknowledged through an identified certification process, in which specific nursing educational requirements and demonstration of knowledge in transplant nursing practice have been delineated and validated (e.g., Certified Clinical Transplant Nurse, Certified Clinical Transplant Coordinator, Certified Procurement Transplant Coordinator).

Transplant nurses may choose to pursue advanced degrees to prepare for advanced transplant nursing practice specialization. Educational requirements vary by specialty, role, educational institution, and country. Upon graduation from an advanced level academic program, transplant nurses may pursue additional certification in a variety of direct and indirect care roles (e.g., clinical nurse specialist, nurse practitioner), based on their educational preparation. In response to changing healthcare, education, and regulatory environments, new models for educational preparation continue to evolve. An advanced certification examination for transplant nursing is a goal for the future.

Knowledge and Skills Base of Transplant Nursing

General transplant nursing care requires a broad knowledge base in anatomy, physiology, immunology, pharmacology, pharmacogenomics, pharmacotherapeutics, nutrition, psychology, sociology, and developmental theory. Clinical competencies beyond those obtained during basic nursing preparation include assessment and management of the deceased transplant donor, assessment and management of the transplant recipient, assessment and management of the potential or living donor, and education and counseling for transplant recipient and living donor related to self-care management, healthy living, and preparation for a peaceful death.

Competencies in serving the physiological, pathophysiological, and psychosocial needs of transplant patients, families, and communities are essential, including skills in helping them age and prepare for death. Transplant nurses must be knowledgeable of the principles of ethical practice and have resources available to evaluate the merits, risks, and social concerns of transplantation. Transplant nurses must be strong advocates for patients, families, and communities of all ages. As transplantation becomes a treatment option for both older and younger patients, transplant nurses must support and advocate for these vulnerable groups.

The core of transplant nursing practice is provision of excellent care based on theory, current evidence, best practices, and consideration of patient preferences using good clinical judgment and decision-making. In providing comprehensive transplant nursing care across the age continuum, the transplant nurse uses the nursing process to assess individual and groups needs, to form an appropriate nursing diagnosis, to design a mutually agreed-on plan of care, to coordinate and provide therapeutic interventions, to document care, and to evaluate this action plan using an interprofessional case management approach.

The transplant nurse also has a global perspective on patient and donor long-term goals, knows the expected clinical course and outcomes in a given transplant situation, and alters plans accordingly. By conducting comprehensive assessments and using analytical abilities and intuition, the transplant nurse operates from a deep understanding of transplant nursing, recognizes when situations are outside the expected, and investigates alternative transplant perspectives. The transplant nurse promotes health and the prevention of injury and disease, serves as a patient and family advocate and educator, provides consultation and education to healthcare providers and the community, and participates in research to improve practice.

Strong assessment skills are the foundation of transplant nursing practice; assessment of transplant rejection and infection is especially critical. Further assessment is related to the specific transplanted organ that the patient has received. For example, if the patient has received a kidney transplant, the transplant nurse will also assess signs and symptoms of decreased urine output related to kidney transplant and knowledge deficit related to dietary and medication modifications post-transplant.

Advances in transplantation include technology for evaluating, monitoring, and treating end-stage organ disease with transplantation. For example, as fetal echocardiography becomes more accurate, earlier diagnosis of high-risk cardiac lesions will be possible with earlier listing for cardiac transplantation (i.e., 36 weeks gestation); implantable artificial hearts are available to prolong life for those waiting for a heart transplant; and transplantation across ABO blood groups is now possible. Transplant nurses accordingly require the knowledge and skills related to these scientific advances.

Many transplant nurses acquire knowledge and skills to use and monitor data from technology used in caring for transplant patients, such as implantable artificial hearts. Transplant nurses use their expertise in these advanced technologies to assess the patient's response to treatment, diagnose the patient's and family's response to the new technology, provide education and support to assist the patient and family to adapt to the new technology, and monitor safety and outcomes. A strong transplant knowledge base is necessary for transplant nurses, administrators, researchers, case managers, transplant coordinators, quality specialists, and educators focused on care of the transplant recipient and donor.

Globalization of Transplant Nursing

Transplant nursing is provided in many countries across the globe. The transplant nurse must consider country-specific issues when caring for transplant patients, families, and communities. These issues are many and varied, and may involve providing transplant nursing care in collaboration with nurses with varied levels of nursing educational preparation. Cultural issues and norms may impact transplantation policies, procedures, availability, and actual transplant care practices. Providing transplant nursing care in countries that have limited financial resources or are involved with selling organs for transplantation may present particularly challenging social and ethical issues for the transplant nurse.

Palliative Care and Transplant Nursing

Palliative care is both a philosophy of care and a system or model for providing care. The goal of palliative care is to prevent or relieve suffering and to focus on helping patients achieve the best possible quality of life throughout their life-limiting or life-threatening illness. The eight recognized domains of palliative care are:

- Structure and process of care,
- Physical aspects of care,
- Psychological aspects of care,
- Social aspects of care,
- Spiritual aspects of care,
- Cultural aspects of care,
- Care of the imminently dying, and
- Ethical or legal aspects of care.

Transplant nursing naturally encompasses many of the palliative care domains, which are reflected in these standards.

Palliative care is ideally implemented early, beginning with diagnosis, and can be provided alongside curative efforts, in an attempt to clarify patient and family goals and preferences, provide aggressive pain and symptom management, offer psychosocial and spiritual support, and address ethical issues.

Transplant nurses are in a unique position to partner with patients and their families as they await transplantation, and then as they manage post-transplant issues, all while implementing the philosophy of palliative care. Should transplantation no longer be an option, or in the event of other post-transplant complications, effective end-of-life (hospice) care, which is one domain of palliative care, will ensure that patients are pain- and symptom-free, and that their goals and wishes are achieved as they live out the best life possible.

Ethics and Informed Decisions

The transplant nurse is concerned about the availability and accessibility of the specialized care required for transplant patients, families, and communities. Transplant nursing is based on the belief that patients and families have the right and responsibility to make informed decisions about their care. The transplant nurse may be faced with caring for patients whose quality of life can be compromised by unanticipated consequences of technological advances in health care. Even as transplant procedures and technologies mature and become more reliable, the potential remains for serious and enduring unanticipated side-effects. Patients and their families and their communities need to know of many such issues.

Ethical issues, situations, and dilemmas unique to the conflicts inherent in transplant nursing may often arise. Transplant recipients and their families face life-threatening illnesses, where survival is dependent on the generosity and suffering of other human beings. Conflicts may arise between the rights of the individual, the rights of families, available accepted scientific and technological treatments, and economic realities. The rights and needs of the potential transplant recipient must be balanced with the rights and needs of the potential donors and their families, whether the donor is living or deceased. There are times when transplantation may no longer be an option as the patient moves along the continuum of life toward death. The transplant nurse is sensitive to palliative care patient and family need and must provide support and comfort at appropriate times.

Because the need for organs greatly exceeds their availability, it is imperative that ethical principles be followed to ensure the fair and equitable distribution of organs. The transplant nurse must be aware of unethical activities such as payment for organs and the trafficking or active selling of organs. The transplant nurse must consider the principles of autonomy, beneficence, confidentiality, equality, and justice when caring for transplant recipients, donors, and families. Of particular importance when caring for living donors is the principle of non-maleficence: to do no harm. At times the rights of individual transplant recipients may appear to conflict with the rights of the donors or with the greater good. The transplant nurse may be involved in the discussions and decision-making to resolve such ethical dilemmas.

The transplant nurse recognizes that each patient is a unique human being, and must protect the individual's basic rights in every phase of the transplant process. The transplant nurse is responsible for reporting incidents of abuse of patients' rights and incompetent, unethical, and illegal practices. In the United States, the transplant nurse should approach ethical decisions as guided by *Code of Ethics for Nurses with Interpretive Statements* (ANA, 2001). This resource may be helpful for transplant nurses in countries where the national professional nurses association does not yet have a code of ethics.

Future Considerations

The specialty of transplant nursing will continue to develop and expand as new technologies and transplant procedures are created to provide healthy tissue and organs to replace those ravaged by cardiovascular disease, diabetes, and related disorders. Efforts to increase the numbers of transplantable organs will remain at the forefront in transplantation. Xenotransplantation—organ transplantation across species—continues to be explored as a way to expand the organ donor pool. Stem cell research will continue to advance the science of creating organs from cells. Composite transplantation—the transplant of tissue such as hand or face tissue from one individual to another—has been successful in several instances. Both extremely young and old patients will receive transplants as technology makes it possible to save more of those who would otherwise die. Using genomics, including pharmocogenomics, to identify patients who would most benefit from transplantation and associated therapies will undoubtedly improve transplant outcomes in the future. Advances in computer technology will allow transplantation to be conducted more effectively and efficiently as information is more readily available and more easily manipulated. Transplant nurses are challenged to remain current through lifelong learning and provide evidenced-based care in this constantly changing environment.

Ethical issues will continue to challenge transplant nurses because some individuals or groups use unethical means to supply organs to those in need, buying organs from vulnerable individuals and marketing the organs to those who can afford them.

The need for transplant nurses is expanding across the world. The aging nursing workforce, coupled with the aging world population, complicates the issue. As the number of specialty nursing areas increases and demand for transplant services mushrooms, transplant administrators are finding it more difficult to attract and retain qualified transplant nurses. This is critical to maintaining and improving transplant patient outcomes. At the same time, the acuity of transplant patients is increasing, and the skills, knowledge, and abilities of transplant nurses currently in transplant nursing must continue to expand correspondingly. Transplant nurses must be active participants in developing and implementing innovative patient care systems and models of care to improve transplant patient care. Nursing education curricula should continue to develop qualified undergraduate and graduate nurses who can specialize in transplantation. As healthcare undergraduate curricula move toward integrated education across professions, transplantation provides a unique opportunity for students and faculty alike to experience integrated teams providing care to patients, families, and communities. Appropriate funding for undergraduate and graduate education must be provided.

The worldwide shortage of physicians provides an opportunity for advanced practice registered nurses to meet the needs of those most vulnerable and in need of care. Advanced practice registered nurses in transplantation can provide the knowledge, experience, and skills to efficiently and effectively fill these healthcare gaps. These nurses are particularly well-positioned to provide chronic illness care to transplant patients, families, and communities and promote effective, preventive self-care and positive outcomes. Healthcare delivery systems designed to support acute episodes of care make it harder to increase desirable long-term patient outcomes. Refocusing the healthcare system on chronic illness and patient self-management can enhance long-term outcomes. Transplant nurses are well-positioned to lead the movement in expanding chronic illness and patient self-management. Advanced practice registered nurses must continue to educate transplant professionals regarding the positive patient outcomes associated with transplant care. They must also work with transplant administrators and regulators to integrate advanced practice registered nurse services into routine transplant health care.

With these changes in health care comes a continued need to emphasize patient safety. Transplant nurses must promote patient, family, and community safety through evidence-based practice and quality improvement efforts. Only through a continuous quest for new knowledge and excellence will transplant nursing excel as a nursing specialty.

STANDARDS OF TRANSPLANT NURSING PRACTICE

Function of Standards

The standards, which are comprised of the standards of practice and the standards of professional performance, are authoritative statements by which nurses practicing within the role, population, and specialty governed by this document (*Nursing Administration: Scope and Standards of Practice*) and that describe the duties that they are expected to competently perform. The standards published herein may be utilized as evidence of the legal standard of care governing nurses practicing within the role, population, and specialty governed by this document. The standards are subject to change with the dynamics of the nursing profession and as new patterns of professional practice are developed and accepted by the nursing profession and the public. In addition, specific conditions and clinical circumstances may also affect the application of the standards at a given time; e.g., during a natural disaster. The standards are subject to formal, periodic review and revision.

The measurement criteria that appear below each standard (pages 24–48) are not all-inclusive and do not establish the legal standard of care. Rather, the measurement criteria are specific, measurable elements that can be used by nursing professionals to measure professional performance. Nurses practicing within this particular role, population, and specialty can identify opportunities for development and improvement by evaluating performance on these elements.

STANDARDS OF PRACTICE

STANDARD 1. ASSESSMENT
The transplant nurse collects comprehensive data pertinent to the patient's health status or situation.

Measurement Criteria:

The transplant nurse:

- Collects clinical data in a systematic and ongoing process.

- Includes the patient, family, and interprofessional healthcare team members in holistic data collection.

- Involves assessment of patients of all ages across the continuum of care from acute to community care.

- Prioritizes data collection based on the patient's immediate condition or anticipated needs.

- Uses developmentally appropriate evidence-based assessment techniques and instruments in data collection.

- Uses analytical models and problem-solving tools.

- Synthesizes data, information, and knowledge relevant to the situation to identify patterns and variances.

- Documents relevant data in a comprehensive and retrievable format.

Additional Measurement Criteria for the Transplant Nurse Coordinator:

The transplant nurse coordinator:

- Initiates diagnostic tests and procedures relative to the transplant patient's current status based on established protocols and procedures.

Additional Measurement Criteria for the Advanced Practice Registered Nurse:

The advanced practice registered nurse:

- Initiates and interprets diagnostic tests and procedures relative to the transplant patient's current status.

STANDARD 2. DIAGNOSIS

The transplant nurse analyzes the assessment data to determine the nursing diagnoses or health-related problems or needs.

Measurement Criteria:

The transplant nurse and transplant nurse coordinator:

- Derives the diagnoses, problems, or needs based on assessment data that reflect the patient's current clinical condition.

- Systematically compares clinical findings with normal and abnormal variations.

- Derives diagnoses encompassing:

  - The patient's identified or potential physical, psychological, social, or developmental problems depending upon the age of the patient.

  - The needs of the child or adolescent to attend school.

  - The needs of the elderly patient regarding integration into post-hospital or long-term care management.

  - The support and educational needs of the family or designated care provider.

  - Any present or potential environmental problem.

- Refines and revises diagnoses regularly based on data subsequently collected.

- Discusses diagnoses, problem, or needs with the patient, family, caregivers, members of the interprofessional team, and other health-care providers when possible and appropriate.

- Documents diagnoses or issues in a manner that facilitates the determination of the expected outcomes and plan.

Continued ▶

Additional Measurement Criteria for the Advanced Practice Registered Nurse:

The advanced practice registered nurse:

- Systematically compares clinical findings with normal and abnormal variations and developmental events in formulating a differential diagnosis.

- Utilizes complex data and information obtained during interview, examination, and diagnostic procedures in identifying diagnoses.

- Assists staff and the interprofessional team in developing and maintaining competency in transplant diagnosis.

STANDARD 3. OUTCOMES IDENTIFICATION
The transplant nurse identifies expected outcomes for a plan individualized to the patient or the situation.

Measurement Criteria:

The transplant nurse:

- Identifies expected outcomes mutually with the patient, family, and other healthcare providers. Expected outcomes are patient-oriented, developmentally appropriate, evidence-based, attainable, and realistic in relation to the patient's, caregiver's, and family's present and potential abilities.

- Derives culturally and age-appropriate expected outcomes from the diagnoses.

- Considers associated risks, benefits, costs, current scientific evidence, and clinical expertise when formulating expected outcomes.

- Defines expected outcomes in terms of the patient, patient values, ethical considerations, environment or situation with consideration of associated risks, benefits and costs, and current scientific evidence.

- Includes a time estimate for attainment of expected outcomes.

- Develops expected outcomes that provide direction for continuity of care.

- Modifies expected outcomes based on patient changes and evaluation of the situation.

- Documents expected outcomes as measurable goals.

- Implements consensus-driven clinical guidelines.

Continued ▶

Additional Measurement Criteria for the Transplant Nurse Coordinator or Advanced Practice Registered Nurse:

The transplant nurse coordinator or advanced practice registered nurse:

- Identifies expected outcomes that incorporate scientific evidence and are achievable through evidence-based practices.

- Identifies expected outcomes that incorporate cost and clinical effectiveness, patient satisfaction, and continuity and consistency among providers.

- Supports the use of clinical guidelines linked to positive patient outcomes.

STANDARD 4. PLANNING
The transplant nurse develops a plan of care that prescribes strategies and alternatives to attain expected outcomes.

Measurement Criteria:

The transplant nurse and transplant nurse coordinator:

- Develops an individualized transplant plan of care that considers patient characteristics, developmental level, and situation (e.g., age- and culturally appropriate, environmentally sensitive).

- Participates in the design and development of interprofessional processes to address the situation or issue.

- Contributes to the development and continuous improvement of organizational systems that support the planning process.

- Supports the integration of clinical, human, and financial resources to enhance and complete the decision-making process.

- Develops the plan in conjunction with the patient, family, and others, synthesizing the patient's values and beliefs, developmental level, and coping style.

- Includes strategies in the plan that address each of the identified diagnoses or issues, which may include strategies for promotion and restoration of health and prevention of illness, injury, and disease.

- Provides for continuity in the plan.

- Incorporates a clinical pathway or timeline in the plan.

- Establishes the plan priorities with the patient, family, and others, as appropriate.

- Utilizes the plan to provide direction to other members of the health-care team.

- Defines the plan to reflect current statutes, rules, regulations, and standards of transplant nursing practice.

- Integrates current trends and research affecting care in planning.

- Considers the economic impact of the plan on the patient, family, caregivers, or other affected parties.

- Uses standardized language or recognized terminology to document the plan.

Continued ▶

Additional Measurement Criteria for the Advanced Practice Registered Nurse:

The advanced practice registered nurse:

- Identifies assessment, diagnostic strategies, and therapeutic interventions in the plan that reflect current evidence, including data, research, literature, and expert clinical knowledge.

- Selects and designs strategies that meet the multifaceted needs of complex transplant patients.

- Includes the synthesis of the patient's values and beliefs regarding nursing and medical therapies in the plan.

STANDARD 5. IMPLEMENTATION
The transplant nurse implements the identified plan.

Measurement Criteria:

The transplant nurse:

- Implements the plan in a safe and timely manner.
- Implements the plan using principles and concepts of project or systems management.
- Fosters organizational systems that support implementation of the plan.
- Documents implementation and any modifications, including changes or omissions, of the identified plan.
- Utilizes evidence-based interventions and treatments specific to the diagnosis or problem.
- Utilizes community resources and systems to implement the plan.
- Collaborates with nursing colleagues and other disciplines to implement the plan.

Additional Measurement Criteria for the Transplant Nurse Coordinator or Advanced Practice Registered Nurse:

The transplant nurse coordinator or advanced practice registered nurse:

- Facilitates utilization of systems and community resources to implement the plan.
- Supports collaboration with nurses and the interprofessional team to implement the plan.
- Incorporates new knowledge and strategies to initiate change in nursing care practices to achieve the desired outcomes.

STANDARD 5A. COORDINATION OF CARE
The transplant nurse coordinates care delivery.

Measurement Criteria:

The transplant nurse:

- Coordinates implementation of the plan.

- Documents coordination of care.

Additional Measurement Criteria for the Transplant Nurse Coordinator or Advanced Practice Registered Nurse:

The transplant nurse coordinator or advanced practice registered nurse:

- Provides leadership in the coordination of the interprofessional healthcare services for the integrated delivery of patient care.

- Synthesizes data and information to facilitate necessary system and community support measures, including environmental modifications.

- Coordinates system and community resources that enhance delivery of care across the continuum.

STANDARD 5B. HEALTH TEACHING AND HEALTH PROMOTION
The transplant nurse employs strategies to promote health and a safe environment.

Measurement Criteria:

The transplant nurse:

- Provides health teaching that addresses such topics as patient self-monitoring, developmental needs, healthy behaviors, activities of daily living, and preventive self-care.

- Uses health promotion and teaching methods appropriate to the situation and the patient's developmental level, learning needs, readiness, ability to learn, literacy level, language preference, and culture.

- Seeks opportunities for feedback and evaluation of the effectiveness of the strategies used.

Additional Measurement Criteria for the Transplant Nurse Coordinator:

The transplant nurse coordinator:

- Designs transplant patient education appropriate to the patient's developmental level, learning needs, readiness to learn, cultural values, and beliefs.

- Designs programs of transplant community education on organ donation, transplantation, and treatment of end-stage organ disease.

Additional Measurement Criteria for the Advanced Practice Registered Nurse:

The advanced practice registered nurse:

- Synthesizes empirical evidence regarding risk behaviors, learning theories, behavioral change and motivational theories, epidemiology, and other related theories when designing health information and patient education.

- Designs transplant patient education appropriate to the patient's developmental level, learning needs, readiness to learn, cultural values, and beliefs.

- Evaluates health information resources such as the Internet in the field of transplantation for accuracy, readability, and comprehensibility to help patients access quality health information.

STANDARD 5C. CONSULTATION

The transplant nurse coordinator or advanced practice registered nurse provides consultation to influence the plan of care, enhance the abilities of others, and effect changes.

Measurement Criteria for the Transplant Nurse Coordinator or Advanced Practice Registered Nurse:

The transplant nurse coordinator or advanced practice registered nurse:

- Synthesizes clinical data, theoretical frameworks, and evidence when providing consultation.

- Facilitates the effectiveness of consultation by involving the patient in decision-making and negotiating role responsibilities.

- Facilitates the effectiveness of a consultation by conducting research and disseminating research findings to enhance psychosocial and clinical outcomes.

- Communicates consultation recommendations to facilitate change.

Standard 5d. Prescriptive Authority and Treatment
The advanced practice registered nurse uses prescriptive authority, procedures, referrals, treatments, and therapies in accordance with state and national laws and regulations.

Measurement Criteria for the Advanced Practice Registered Nurse:

The advanced practice registered nurse:

• Prescribes evidence-based treatments, therapies, and procedures considering the patient's comprehensive healthcare needs.

• Prescribes pharmacologic agents based on a current knowledge of pharmacology and physiology.

• Prescribes specific pharmacological agents and treatments based on clinical indicators, the patient's status and needs, and the results of diagnostic and laboratory tests.

• Evaluates therapeutic and potential adverse effects of pharmacological and non-pharmacological treatments.

• Provides patients with information about intended effects and potential adverse effects of proposed prescriptive therapies.

• Provides information about costs, alternative treatments, and procedures, as appropriate.

STANDARD 6. EVALUATION

The transplant nurse evaluates progress towards attainment of outcomes.

Measurement Criteria:

The transplant nurse:

- Conducts a systematic, ongoing, and criterion-based evaluation of the outcomes in relation to the structure and processes prescribed by the plan and the indicated timeline.

- Includes the patient and others involved in the care or situation in the evaluative process.

- Evaluates the effectiveness of the planned strategies in relation to patient responses and the attainment of the expected outcomes.

- Documents results of the evaluation.

- Uses ongoing assessment data to revise the diagnoses, outcomes, the plan, and the implementation as needed.

- Synthesizes the results of the evaluation to determine the impact of the plan on the affected patients, families, groups, communities, institutions, networks, and organizations.

- Disseminates the results to the patient and others involved in the care or situation, as appropriate, in accordance with country and state laws and regulations.

Additional Measurement Criteria for the Transplant Nurse Coordinator or Advanced Practice Registered Nurse:

The transplant nurse coordinator or advanced practice registered nurse:

- Evaluates the accuracy of the diagnosis and effectiveness of the interventions in relation to the patient's attainment of expected outcomes.

- Uses the results of the evaluation to make or recommend process or structure changes, including policy, procedure, or protocol documentation, as appropriate.

STANDARDS OF PROFESSIONAL PERFORMANCE

STANDARD 7. QUALITY OF PRACTICE
The transplant nurse systematically enhances the quality and effectiveness of nursing practice.

Measurement Criteria:

The transplant nurse:

- Demonstrates quality by documenting the application of the nursing process in a responsible, accountable, and ethical manner.

- Uses the results of quality improvement activities to initiate changes in nursing practice and in the healthcare delivery system.

- Uses creativity and innovation in nursing practice to improve care delivery.

- Incorporates new knowledge to initiate changes in nursing practice if desired outcomes are not achieved.

- Obtains and maintains professional certification.

- Designs quality improvement initiatives.

- Implements initiatives to evaluate the need for change.

- Evaluates the practice environment in relation to existing evidence, identifying opportunities for the generation and use of research.

- Participates in quality improvement activities. Such activities may include:

  - Identifying aspects of practice important for quality monitoring.

  - Using indicators developed to monitor quality and effectiveness of nursing practice.

  - Collecting data to monitor quality and effectiveness of nursing practice.

  - Analyzing quality data to identify opportunities for improving nursing practice.

Continued ▶

- Formulating recommendations to improve nursing practice or outcomes.

- Implementing activities to enhance the quality of nursing practice.

- Developing, implementing, and evaluating policies, procedures and guidelines to improve the quality of practice.

- Participating on interprofessional teams to evaluate clinical care or health services.

- Participating in efforts to minimize costs and unnecessary duplication.

- Analyzing factors related to safety, satisfaction, effectiveness, and cost–benefit options.

- Analyzing organizational systems for barriers.

- Implementing processes to remove or decrease barriers within organizational systems.

STANDARD 8. EDUCATION

The transplant nurse attains knowledge and competency that reflects current nursing practice.

Measurement Criteria:

The transplant nurse:

- Participates in ongoing educational activities related to appropriate knowledge bases and professional issues.

- Demonstrates a commitment to lifelong learning through self-reflection and inquiry to identify learning needs.

- Seeks experiences that reflect current practice in order to maintain skills and competence in clinical practice or role performance.

- Acquires knowledge and skills appropriate to the specialty area, practice setting, role, or situation.

- Maintains professional records that provide evidence of competency and lifelong learning.

- Seeks formal and independent learning activities, and experiences to maintain and develop clinical and professional skills and knowledge.

- Uses current healthcare research findings and other evidence to expand clinical knowledge, enhance role performance, and increase knowledge of professional issues.

- Obtains and maintains professional certification.

STANDARD 9. PROFESSIONAL PRACTICE EVALUATION

The transplant nurse evaluates one's own nursing practice in relation to professional practice standards and guidelines, relevant statutes, rules, and regulations.

Measurement Criteria:

The transplant nurse:

- Applies knowledge of current practice standards, guidelines, statutes, rules, and regulations into practice.

- Provides age- and developmentally appropriate care in a culturally and ethnically sensitive manner.

- Engages in self-evaluation of practice on a regular basis, identifying areas of strength as well as areas in which professional development would be beneficial.

- Obtains informal feedback regarding one's own practice from patients, peers, professional colleagues, and others.

- Participates in systematic peer review as appropriate.

- Takes action to achieve goals identified during the evaluation process.

- Provides rationales for practice beliefs, decisions, and actions as part of the informal and formal evaluation processes.

- Engages in a formal process seeking feedback regarding role performance from individuals, professional colleagues, representatives, administrators of corporate entities, and others.

STANDARD 10. COLLEGIALITY

The transplant nurse interacts with, and contributes to the professional development of, peers, colleagues, and others.

Measurement Criteria:

The transplant nurse:

- Shares knowledge and skills with peers and colleagues as evidenced by such activities as patient care conferences or presentation at formal or informal meetings.

- Provides peers with feedback regarding their practice or role performance.

- Interacts with peers and colleagues to enhance one's own professional nursing practice and role performance.

- Maintains compassionate and caring relationships with peers and colleagues.

- Supports and facilitates education of students in healthcare professions.

- Contributes to a supportive and healthy work environment.

- Actively participates on multiprofessional teams that contribute to role development and, directly and indirectly, advance nursing practice and health services.

- Mentors other registered nurses and colleagues as appropriate.

Additional Measurement Criteria for the Transplant Nurse Coordinator or Advanced Practice Registered Nurse:

The transplant nurse coordinator or advanced practice registered nurse:

- Models expert practice to interprofessional team members and healthcare consumers.

STANDARD 11. COLLABORATION

The transplant nurse collaborates with patients, family, and others in the conduct of nursing practice.

Measurement Criteria:

The transplant nurse:

- Communicates with the patient, family, and healthcare providers regarding patient care and the nurse's role in providing that care.

- Collaborates in creating a documented plan focused on outcomes and decisions related to care and delivery of services that indicates communication with patients, families, and others.

- Consults with other disciplines to enhance patient care through interprofessional activities such as education, consultation, management, technological development, or research opportunities.

- Partners with others to effect change and generate positive outcomes through knowledge of the patient or situation.

- Documents referrals, including provisions for continuity of care.

Additional Measurement Criteria for the Transplant Nurse Coordinator or Advanced Practice Registered Nurse:

The transplant nurse coordinator or advanced practice registered nurse:

- Partners with other disciplines to enhance patient care through interprofessional activities, such as education, consultation, management, technology development, or research activities.

- Facilitates an interprofessional process with other members of the healthcare team.

- Documents plan-of-care communications, rationales for plan-of-care changes, and collaborative discussions to improve patient care.

STANDARD 12. ETHICS

The transplant nurse integrates ethical principles in all areas of practice.

Measurement Criteria:

The transplant nurse:

- Uses *Code of Ethics for Nurses with Interpretive Statements* (ANA, 2001) to guide practice.

- Delivers care in a manner that preserves and protects patient autonomy, dignity, and rights.

- Maintains patient confidentiality within legal and regulatory parameters.

- Serves as a patient advocates assisting patients in developing skills for self-advocacy.

- Maintains a therapeutic and professional patient–nurse relationship within appropriate professional role boundaries.

- Demonstrates a commitment to practicing self-care, managing stress, and connecting with self and others.

- Contributes to resolving ethical issues of patients, colleagues, or systems as evidenced by such activities as participating on ethics committees.

- Reports illegal, incompetent, or impaired practices.

- Informs patients of the risks, benefits, and outcomes of healthcare regimens.

- Participates in interprofessional teams that address ethical risks, benefits, and outcomes.

Additional Measurement Criteria for the Advanced Practice Registered Nurse:

The advanced practice registered nurse:

- Develops or facilitates nursing research related to ethical issues that emerge during patient care experiences.

STANDARD 13. RESEARCH
The transplant nurse integrates research findings into practice.

Measurement Criteria:

The transplant nurse:

- Utilizes the best available evidence, including research findings, to guide practice decisions.

- Actively participates in research activities at various levels appropriate to the nurse's level of education and position. Activities may include:

  - Identifying clinical problems specific to nursing research (patient care and nursing practice).

  - Participating in data collection (surveys, pilot projects, and formal studies).

  - Participating in a formal committee or program.

  - Sharing research activities and findings with peers and others.

  - Conducting research.

  - Critically analyzing and interpreting research for application to practice.

  - Using research findings in the development of policies, procedures, and standards of practice in patient care.

  - Incorporating research as a basis for learning.

- Participates in human subject protection activities as appropriate, and is particularly cognizant of the needs of the transplant group served.

Additional Measurement Criteria for the Advanced Practice Registered Nurse:

The advanced practice registered nurse:

- Contributes to nursing knowledge by conducting or synthesizing research that discovers, examines, and evaluates knowledge, theories, criteria, and creative approaches to improve health care.

- Formally disseminates research findings through activities such as presentations, publications, consultation, and journal clubs.

- Mentors transplant nurses in conducting and evaluating transplant nursing research.

STANDARD 14. RESOURCE UTILIZATION

The transplant nurse considers factors related to safety, effectiveness, cost, and impact on practice in the planning and delivery of nursing services.

Measurement Criteria:

The transplant nurse:

- Uses organizational and community resources to formulate interprofessional plans of care.

- Evaluates factors such as safety, effectiveness, availability, cost–benefits, efficiencies, and impact on practice, when choosing among practice options that would result in the same expected outcome.

- Assists the patient and family in identifying and securing appropriate and available services to address health-related needs.

- Assigns or delegates tasks, based on the needs and condition of the patient, potential for harm, stability of the patient's condition, complexity of the task, and predictability of the outcome.

- Assists the patient and family in becoming informed consumers about the options, costs, risks, and benefits of treatment and care.

Additional Measurement Criteria for the Transplant Nurse Coordinator or Advanced Practice Registered Nurse:

The transplant nurse coordinator or advanced practice registered nurse:

- Develops innovative solutions for patient care problems that address effective resources utilization and maintenance of quality.

- Uses organizational and community resources to formulate interprofessional plans of care.

- Develops evaluation strategies to demonstrate cost effectiveness, cost benefit, and efficiency factors associated with nursing practice.

- Promotes activities that assist others, as appropriate, in becoming informed about costs, risks, and benefits of care, or of the plan and solution.

STANDARD 15. LEADERSHIP

The transplant nurse provides leadership in the professional practice setting and the profession.

Measurement Criteria:

The transplant nurse:

- Engages in teamwork as a team player and a team builder.

- Works to create and maintain healthy work environments in local, regional, national, or international communities.

- Displays the ability to define a clear vision, the associated goals, and a plan to implement and measure progress.

- Demonstrates a commitment to continuous, lifelong learning for self and others.

- Teaches others to succeed by mentoring and other strategies.

- Exhibits creativity and flexibility through times of change.

- Demonstrates energy, excitement, and a passion for quality work.

- Willingly accepts mistakes by self and others, thereby creating a culture in which risk-taking is not only safe, but expected.

- Inspires loyalty by valuing people as the most precious asset in an organization.

- Directs the coordination of care across settings and among caregivers or providers, including oversight of licensed and unlicensed personnel in any assigned or delegated tasks.

- Serves in key roles in the work setting by participating on committees, councils, and administrative teams.

- Promotes advancement of the profession through participation in professional organizations.

Continued ▶

Additional Measurement Criteria for the Transplant Nurse Coordinator or Advanced Practice Registered Nurse:

The transplant nurse coordinator or advanced practice registered nurse:

- Works to influence decision-making bodies to improve patient care.

- Provides direction to enhance the effectiveness of the healthcare team.

- Initiates and revises protocols or guidelines to reflect evidence-based practice, incorporate accepted changes in care management, or solve emerging problems.

- Promotes communication of information and advancement of the profession through writing, publishing, and presentations for professionals or lay audiences.

- Designs innovations to effect change in practice and outcomes.

Glossary

Assessment. A systematic, dynamic process by which the nurse, through interaction with the patient, significant others, and healthcare providers, collects and analyzes data about the patient. Data may include the following dimensions: physical, psychological, sociocultural, spiritual, cognitive, functional, developmental, economic, and lifestyle.

Caregiver. A person who provides direct care for another, such as a child, dependent adult, the disabled, or the chronically ill.

Code of ethics. A list of provisions that makes explicit the primary goals, values, and obligations of the profession.

Continuity of care. An interprofessional process that includes patients and significant others in the development of a coordinated plan of care. This process facilitates the patient's transition between settings, based on changing needs and available resources.

Criteria. Relevant, measurable indicators of the standards of clinical nursing practice.

Data. Discrete entities that are described objectively without interpretation.

Diagnosis. A clinical judgment about the patient's response to actual or potential health conditions or needs. The diagnosis provides the basis for determination of a plan of care to achieve expected outcomes. Transplant nurses utilize nursing or medical diagnoses depending upon educational and clinical preparation and legal authority.

Disease. A biological or psychosocial disorder of structure or function in a patient, especially one that produces specific signs or symptoms or that affects a specific part of the body, mind, or spirit.

Environment. The atmosphere, milieu, or conditions in which an individual lives, works, or plays.

Evaluation. The process of determining both the patient's progress toward the attainment of expected outcomes and the effectiveness of nursing care.

Evidence-based practice. A process founded on the collection, interpretation, and integration of valid, important, and applicable patient-reported, clinician-observed, or research-derived evidence. The best available evidence, moderated by patient circumstances and preferences, is applied to improve the quality of clinical judgments.

Expected outcomes. End results that are measurable, desirable, and observable, and that translate into observable behaviors.

Family. Family of origin or significant others as identified by the patient.

Guidelines. Systematic statements, based on available scientific evidence and expert opinion, that describe a process of patient care management which has the potential to improve the quality of clinical and consumer decision-making.

Health. "A state of complete physical, mental and social well-being and not merely the absence of disease or infirmity" (WHO, 1946).

Healthcare provider. A person with special expertise who provides healthcare services or assistance to patients. This may include nurses, physicians, psychologists, social workers, nutritionist/dietitians, and various therapists.

Holistic. Based on an understanding that the patient is an interconnected unity, a whole system that is greater than the sum of its parts, and that physical, mental, social, and spiritual factors need to be included in any interventions.

Hospice care. The provision of palliative care for patients who are in the terminal stages of illness, with an emphasis on biomedical, psychosocial, and spiritual support. Hospice care supports family members, and addresses the bereavement needs of the family following the death of the patient (National Consensus Project for Quality Palliative Care, 2004).

Illness. The subjective experience of discomfort.

Implementation. Activities such as teaching, monitoring, providing, counseling, delegating, and coordinating. The patient, significant others, or healthcare providers may be designated to implement interventions within the plan of care.

Information. Data that are interpreted, organized, or structured.

Interprofessional. Reliant on the overlapping knowledge, skills, and abilities of each professional team member, resulting in synergistic effects where outcomes are enhanced and more comprehensive than the simple aggregation of the team members' individual efforts.

Knowledge. Information that is synthesized so that relationships are identified and formalized.

Nurse. An adequately educated and prepared individual registered or licensed by a state, commonwealth, territory, government, or other regulatory body to practice as a registered nurse.

Nursing. The diagnosis and treatment of human responses to actual or potential health behaviors.

Outcomes. Measurable, expected, patient-focused goals that translate into observable behaviors.

Palliative care. Patient- and family-centered care focused on the prevention or relief of pain and suffering, and on maximizing quality of life. Palliative care is provided throughout the course of a life-threatening or life-limiting illness by an interprofessional team in order to ensure comprehensive assessment and management of the patient's medical, psychosocial, and spiritual needs (National Consensus Project for Quality Palliative Care, 2004).

Patient. Recipient of transplant nursing care, whether the potential deceased or potential living donor, the deceased or living donor, and the transplant recipient. When an individual, the focus is on his or her health state, problems, or needs. When a family or group, the focus is on their health state as a whole or the reciprocal effects of an individual's health state on the others. When a community or population, the focus is on their collective personal and environmental health and the health risks.

Peer review. A collegial, systematic, and periodic process by which registered nurses are held accountable for practice and which fosters the refinement of knowledge, skills, and decision-making at all levels and in all areas of practice.

Plan. A comprehensive outline of the steps that need to be undertaken to attain expected outcomes.

Quality of care. The degree to which health services for patients increase the likelihood of desired health outcomes, and are consistent with current professional knowledge.

Quality of life. An individual's general perception of happiness and satisfaction with life; domains include health, physical, psychological, financial, social, family, economic, and spiritual areas. The transplant patient's perception may focus on health-related quality of life issues, and the impact on his or her normal functioning by disease or illness.

Recipients of nursing care. *See* Patient

Self-care maintenance. Self-monitoring adherence behaviors used by patients to maintain health.

Self-care management. The decision-making process that patients use when conducting self-care maintenance.

Situation. A set of circumstances, conditions, or events.

Standard. An authoritative statement enunciated and promulgated by the profession, by which the quality of practice, service or education can be judged.

Standards of nursing care. Authoritative statements that describe a competent level of clinical nursing practice demonstrated through assessment, diagnosis, outcomes identification, planning, implementation, and evaluation.

Standards of practice. Authoritative statements that describe a level of care or performance common to the profession of nursing by which the quality of nursing practice can be judged. Standards of clinical nursing practice include both standards of care and standards of professional performance.

Standards of professional performance. Authoritative statements that describe a competent level of behavior in the professional role, including quality of care, professional practice evaluation, education, collegiality, ethics, collaboration, research, resource utilization, and leadership.

Strategy. A plan of action to achieve a major overall goal.

Transplant nursing. Specialized nursing care of the transplant recipient and donor with these foci:

- Protection, promotion, and optimization of health and abilities of the transplant recipient and living donor across the life span. Includes prevention, detection, and treatment of illness and injury related to diseases treated by solid organ transplantation, and diseases that may occur due to living donor donation in individuals, families, communities, and populations of all ages.

- Protection, promotion, and optimization of the deceased organ donor during the process of organ donation. Includes prevention, detection, and treatment of illness and injury that may occur during the process of organ donation and recovery in individuals and families of all ages.

REFERENCES

American Nurses Association (ANA). (2001). *Code of ethics for nurses with interpretive statements.* Silver Spring, MD: Nursesbooks.org.

American Nurses Association (ANA). (2004). *Nursing: Scope and standards of practice.* Silver Spring, MD: Nursesbooks.org.

Galbraith, C. A., & Hathaway, D. (2004). Long-term effects of transplantation on quality of life. *Transplantation, 77*(9 Suppl), S84–S87.

Institute of Medicine (IOM). (2001). *Crossing the quality chasm: A new health system for the 21st century.* Washington, DC: National Academies Press.

International Council of Nurses (ICN). (2002). *ICN announces position on advanced nursing roles.* Retrieved April 23, 2009 from http://www.icn.ch/PR19_02.htm

National Association of Clinical Nurse Specialists (NACNS). (2004). *Statement on clinical nurse specialist practice and education.*

National Consensus Project for Quality Palliative Care. (2004). *Clinical practice guidelines for quality palliative care.* Retrieved April 23, 2009 from http://www.nationalconsensusproject.org/Guideline.pdf

United Network for Organ Sharing (UNOS). (2008). Retrieved April 23, 2009 from http://www.unos.org

World Health Organization (WHO). (1946). Retrieved April 23, 2009 from http://www.who.int/suggestions/faq/en/

Index

Collaboration (*continued*)
 transplant nurse coordinator, 10–11
 See also Interprofessional teams in
  transplant nursing care
Collegiality
 peer review and, 40
 standard of professional performance,
  41
Communities and transplant care, 3, 21
 education of, 2, 4
 nurse advocacy for, 9, 14, 17
 organ donations and, 7
Competence assessment. *See* Certification
  and credentialing
Competence and competencies, 15, 16,
  39
 diagnosis standard and, 26
 education standard and, 39
 See also Certification and
  credentialing
Confidentiality. *See* Ethics
Conflict management in
  transplantation, 19–20
 See also Ethics
Consultation, 14
 standard of practice, 34
Continuity of care
 defined, 49
 documentation of, 42
 outcomes identification and, 27
Coordination of care, 5
 standard of practice, 32
Cost controls in transplant care, 11, 14,
  27, 28, 35
Credentialing. *See* Certification and
  credentialing
Criteria for standards (measurement
  criteria)
 assessment, 24
 collaboration, 42
 collegiality, 41
 consultation, 34
 coordination of care, 32
 defined, 49
 diagnosis, 25–26
 education, 39
 ethics, 43

evaluation, 36
health teaching and health promotion,
 33
implementation, 31
leadership, 47–48
outcomes identification, 27–28
planning, 29–30
prescriptive authority and treatment,
 35
professional practice evaluation, 40
quality of practice, 37–38
research, 44–45
resource utilization, 46
Cultural sensitivity in care, 18, 19, 27, 29,
 33, 40

D
Data collection,
 in assessment, 24, 25, 36
 in quality practice, 37
 in research, 44
Data and information analysis, synthesis,
  and use
 APRNs and, 13
 in assessment, 24
 in consulting, 34
 in coordination of care, 32
 defined, 49
 in diagnosis, 25–26
 in evaluation, 36
 in planning, 30
Developmentally appropriate care, 24,
 25, 29, 33, 40
Death and dying. *See* Palliative care
Diagnosis
 assessment data and, 25, 36
 defined, 49
 standard of practice, 25–26
Disease (defined), 49
Documentation
 of assessment data, 24
 collaboration and, 42
 of coordination of care, 32
 of continuity of care, 42
 of diagnosis, 25
 in evaluation, 36
 of expected outcomes, 27

of implementation, 31
in planning, 29, 31, 42
of quality of practice, 37
Donors and transplant care, 2–4
coordination of nursing care for, 5–6, 10–12
education and counseling of, 16–18
ethical issues and conflicts, 19–20
See also Recipients and transplant care

E

Economic issues. *See* Cost controls
Education
certification and, 39
collegiality and, 41
standard of professional performance, 39
transplant nurse, 15–16
Elders as patients, 25
See also Age-appropriate care, Developmentally appropriate care
End of life care. *See* Palliative care
Environment, 25, 27, 32
defined, 49
See also Practice environment
Ethics, 9, 16, 21
globalization of transplantation and, 18
informed decision and, 19–20
organ buyers and, 21
in palliative care, 18–19
quality of practice and, 37
standard of professional performance, 43
See also Code of Ethics with Interpretive Statements
Evaluation
defined, 49
resource utilization and, 46
standard of practice, 36
Evidence-based practice,
defined, 50
transplant nursing and, 4, 5, 9, 14, 21
See also Research
Expected outcomes
defined, 50
diagnosis and, 25

evaluation and 36
identification of, 27–28
plan of care and, 29
resource utilization and, 46
See also Outcomes identification

F

Families as recipients of transplant care, 3, 4, 6, 18, 22
organ donations and, 7
nurse advocacy for, 4, 6, 9, 19, 14
rights of, 19–20
Family (defined), 50

G

Generalist level transplant nursing, 12–13
See also Transplant nursing
Globalization and transplantion, 18
Guidelines
defined, 50
outcomes identification and, 27, 28
in professional performance evaluation, 40
quality of practice and, 37, 38, 48

H

Health (defined), 50
Health teaching and health promotion, 17, 22
clinical nurse specialist, 14–15
nurse practitioners and, 14
standard of practice, 33
Healthcare provider (defined), 50
Holistic (defined), 50
Hospice care (defined), 50
See also Palliative care

I

Illness (defined), 50
Implementation
coordination of care and, 32
defined, 50
standard of practice, 31
Information (defined), 50
Information analysis, synthesis, and use. *See* Data and information analysis, synthesis, and use

Informed decisions and ethics, 19–20
International aspects of transplant
    nursing, 12, 13
International Transplant Nurses Society
    (ITNS), 4, 8–9
Interprofessional (defined), 51
Interprofessional teams in transplant
    nursing care, 2, 8, 9, 14, 17
    continuity of care and, 49
    coordination of care and, 32
    data collection and, 24
    diagnosis and, 25, 26
    ethics and, 43
    implementation and, 31
    planning and, 29, 46
    quality of practice and, 38
    resource utilization and, 46

K
Knowledge (defined), 51
Knowledge base of transplant nursing,
    3, 4, 7–8, 16–17, 18, 21–22, 39
    advanced practice transplant nurses
    and, 12–13

L
Leadership, standard of professional
    performance, 47–48
Levels of practice. *See* Advanced
    practice registered nurse (APRN);
    Generalist level transplant nursing
Licensing, 10, 12, 15
    See also Certification and
    credentialing
Living donor nurse coordinator
    collaboration, 10, 11
    practice settings and roles, 6
    role differentiation, 10, 11
Living donors. *See* Donors and transplant
    care

M
Measurement criteria. *See* Criteria for
    standards

N
Nurse (defined), 51

Nurse coordinator. *See* Transplant nurse
    coordinator
Nurse practitioner (NP), 13–14
Nursing (defined), 51
Nursing process in transplant nursing
    practice, 17
    and quality of practice, 37
Nursing standards. *See* Standards of
    practice…; Standards of
    professional performance…

O
Organ (solid) transplantation, 2–3
    See also Procurement of organs;
    Transplant organs
Organization systems in transplant
    nursing, 29, 31, 36, 38
Organizations. *See* Professional
    organizations in transplant
    nursing
Outcomes
    defined, 51
    optimization of in transplant care,
    4, 7, 11
    See also Expected outcomes
Outcomes identification
    as identification of expected out-
    comes, 27
    standard of practice, 27–28
    See also Expected outcomes

P
Palliative care
    defined, 51
    transplant nursing and, 18–19
Parents. *See* Family; Families …
Patients
    defined, 51
    post-transplant care, 11–12
    pre-transplant care, 11–12
    See also Communities and transplant
    care; Donors and transplant care;
    Families as patients in transplant
    care; Recipients of nursing and
    transplant care
Peer review, 40
    defined, 51

knowledge and skills base, 16–18
overview, 2–4
palliative care and, 18–19
practice settings and roles, 5–6
research, 5
trends and future of, 20–22
Transplant organs, 2–3
availability of, 2
education of donors, 7, 11
end-stage diseases, 18

ethics and procurement, 21
Transplant recipients. *See* Recipients of
transplant care

W
Work environment. *See* Practice
environments

X
Xenotransplantation, 21